Pocket Picture Guides

Fungal Nail Infection

The illustrations on the cover show the four types of fungal
infection of the nails (from top left, clockwise):
  Distal and lateral subungual onychomycosis (DLSO)
  Proximal subungual onychomycosis (PSO)
  Total dystrophic onychomycosis (TDO)
  Superficial white onychomycosis (SWO).

Pocket Picture Guides

Fungal Nail Infection

D.T. Roberts
MB, ChB, FRCP (Glas)
Consultant Dermatologist
Southern General Hospital and Victoria Infirmary
Glasgow

E.G.V. Evans
BSc, PhD, MIBiol
Senior Lecturer in Medical Mycology
University of Leeds and General Infirmary
Leeds

B.R. Allen
MB, ChB, FRCP (Lond)
Consultant Dermatologist
University Hospital
Queens Medical Centre
Nottingham

Produced and published by Gower Medical Publishing

ISBN 0-397-44780-9

Printed in Italy by L.E.G.O. Vicenza 1990. Reprinted 1991.

Contents

Picture Credits viii

Acknowledgements....................................ix

1. Introduction..................................... ..,,......1

2. Nail Structure 3
    Points to note...6

3. Types of Abnormality............................7
    Longitudinal ridging.....................................8
    Transverse ridging.......................................11
    Transverse layering or lamellar nail splitting ...14
    Thickening of the nail 15
    Separation of the nail plate 18
    Discolouration..21

Inflammation of the nail fold..............................28

Painful nails...33

Pitting 36

Other abnormalities 37

Points to note...40

4. Fungal Nail Disease...............................41

Clinical features 42

Points to note...47

5. Mycology and Epidemiology..............49

The fungi...49

Pathogens of nails..51

Dermatophytes 51

Other moulds 53

Yeasts...55

Prevalence of fungal nail disease 57

Points to note...59

6. Diagnosis of Fungal Nail Infection 61

Clinical diagnosis 61

Laboratory diagnosis 61

General principles 61

Collection of samples.....................................62

Laboratory procedures 63

Interpretation of results 65

Points to note...68

7. Treatment of Fungal Nail Infections ..69
   Topical treatment...70
   Systemic treatment...72
   New developments in the treatment of fungal
      nail infection...73
   Points to note..76

Conclusion 77

Further Reading 79

Index 80

Picture Credits

The figures illustrating onychogryphosis on page 15 and onycholysis due to psoriasis on page 19 are reproduced from the *Atlas of Clinical Dermatology* by Anthony du Vivier, published by Gower Medical Publishing, London.

The figures showing *Scopulariopsis brevicaulis* on page 64 and *Epidermophyton floccosum* on page 66 are reproduced from the *Pocket Picture Guide to Medical Mycology* by Yvonne Clayton and Gillian Midgley, published by Gower Medical Publishing, London. These figures are copyright of the Institute of Dermatology, UMDS of Guy's and St. Thomas's Hospitals, London.

The figure showing *Hendersonula toruloidea* on page 66 is reproduced courtesy of Mary K. Moore.

Acknowledgements

The Authors wish to acknowledge help, in the provision of illustrations, of the Departments of Dermatology and Medical Illustration at the Western Infirmary, Glasgow; the Royal Hospital for Sick Children, Glasgow; the Southern General Hospital, Glasgow; and the Audio Visual Department at Queen's Medical Centre, Nottingham.

Grateful thanks also to R.A. Forster for his help with the illustrations.

Chapter One

Introduction

The distorted, discoloured or otherwise damaged nail is of mechanical and cosmetic importance to the patient as well as being of diagnostic significance. The integrity of the nail plate can be disturbed by a number of circumstances which may reflect the patient's age, occupation and general health as well as by specific disease of the nail itself.

The main aim of this small book is to discuss the diagnosis and therapy of fungal infection of the nail (onychomycosis). It is important that fungal infections, which can be treated effectively, are correctly diagnosed and differentiated from other nail disorders, the majority of which are irremediable in terms of direct treatment.

Fungal infections are common but there is a tendency for those not experienced in the examination of nails to diagnose almost every abnormality as 'fungal' and to subject the patient to weeks, months or even years of pointless treatment. In order to evaluate properly the patient with possible onychomycosis, it is necessary to relate the nail changes to the structure of normal nail and to those changes seen in other disorders. Dermatophyte infection (dermatophytosis) is the commonest fungal nail disorder and will therefore be given most attention in this book, particularly in view of recent significant developments in therapy. However, other fungi can and do attack nails and are not always amenable to the same treatment, thus they must be differentiated from dermatophytes.

Chapter Two

Nail Structure

Some knowledge of the structure and property of normal nail is necessary in order to appreciate the patterns of change seen in nail disease; the basic anatomy of normal nail is illustrated in **Figure 1**.

The nail plate consists of keratin formed by flattening of the keratinocytes of the matrix followed by fragmentation of their nuclei and condensation of the cell

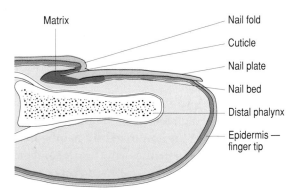

Figure 1. Structure of the nail

cytoplasm to form a flat, compact, horny layer. The matrix extends forward from beneath the proximal nail fold and is delineated by the lunula or 'half moon' which marks its distal end. About one quarter of the nail is beneath the nail fold and the exposed part is attached to the nail bed which has a profuse blood supply thus providing the nail with its pink colour. The tip of the nail which is not attached to the nail bed is an opaque white colour and this can extend down the nail if it becomes detached from the bed, a condition known as onycholysis.

The nail fold is attached to the nail plate via the cuticle, which is watertight. When the cuticle becomes detached from the nail plate its waterproof properties are lost allowing various organisms and irritants to wash under it and potentially setting up infection or irritation in the area of the matrix. The nail fold swells in such circumstances, detaching the cuticle even further and a vicious circle of infection and inflammation is set up. This is known as chronic paronychia and it will ultimately destroy the nail plate proximally.

Some fungi, notably, *Candida*, enter the nail by this route but the portal of entry of dermatophyte fungi, the main pathogens of nails, is through the distal and lateral undersurface.

The nail bed is supplied with blood by arches derived from the digital arteries **(Figure 2)**. Arteriovenous connections are controlled by neurovascular bundles called glomus bodies which can sometimes be the seat of small tumours called glomus tumours. It has long been believed that drugs only reach the nail by incorporation into the keratin as the nail grows but it has been shown recently that this is untrue. It is now thought that the blood supply to the nail bed allows drugs to diffuse upwards into all parts of the nail and not, as previously believed, only into the proximal area of the matrix. Therefore antifungal drugs arrive at the nailtip in adequate concentration within a few weeks of the start of treatment; a consideration which is likely to be important in terms of length of therapy with the newer antifungal drugs.

In addition to keratin the rigid structure of nail contains numerous trace minerals. Calcium is found in moderate concentration but there is little evidence to support the widely held belief that it contributes directly to nail hardness.

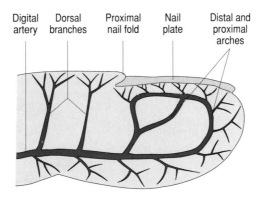

Figure 2. Blood supply of the nail

NAIL STRUCTURE

POINTS TO NOTE

l. Nail itself is translucent. The pink colour is provided by the nail bed and will change to white whenever the nail becomes detached from the bed.

2. The cuticle must remain attached to the nail plate to keep it waterproof.

3. Antifungal drugs can probably diffuse into the whole length of the nail simultaneously.

Chapter Three

Types of Abnormality

Nail disease can affect just the nail plate or the peri-onychial tissues or both. The disorders which involve the nail plate may alter nail configuration, modify the nail surface or lead to colour change. Common physical signs which are often confused with fungal infection are listed in **Table 1**. Other well recognised abnormalities are less frequently mistaken for fungal nail disease and therefore are not discussed in detail.

Table 1. Common physical signs which are often confused with fungal infection of the nail

PHYSICAL SIGNS OFTEN CONFUSED WITH FUNGAL INFECTION OF THE NAIL
Longitudinal ridging
Transverse ridging
Transverse layering and splitting
Thickening of the nail
Separation of the nail plate
Discolouration
Inflammation around the nail fold
Painful nails
Pitting

Longitudinal Ridging

LONGITUDINAL RIDGING	
Physical signs	**Underlying causes**
Shallow parallel furrows	Age Twenty nail dystrophy Lichen planus Rheumatoid arthritis Peripheral circulatory disorders Several genetic diseases
Deeper parallel furrows	Lichen planus Alopecia areata Darier's disease Trauma
Deep wide longitudinal groove	Tumours eg. myxoid cysts and warts
Single longitudinal defect usually in thumb nail	Median nail dystrophy

Shallow parallel furrows separated by low ridges are physiological and become more prominent with age. They can also occur to a pathological degree in twenty nail dystrophy, lichen planus, rheumatoid arthritis, peripheral circulatory disorders and several genetic diseases.

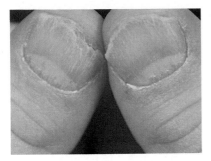

Shallow parallel furrows in twenty nail dystrophy

Deeper parallel furrows can become discoloured by ingrained dirt and may be severe enough to result in splitting of the free edge of the nail. They may be seen in lichen planus, alopecia areata, Darier's disease and trauma.

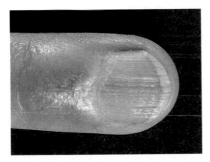

Longitudinal ridging due to lichen planus

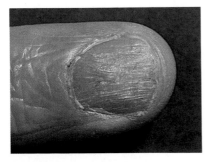

Alopecia areata affecting the nail

Tumours such as **myxoid cysts** and **warts** located in the proximal nail fold sometimes exert pressure on the matrix and produce a deep, wide longitudinal groove which is usually single. If the cause can be removed without further damage to the nail matrix the abnormality will resolve.

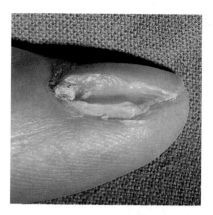

Deep wide longitudinal groove due to fibroma

Median nail dystrophy is an uncommon condition of unknown aetiology, consisting of a single longitudinal defect, which nearly always affects both thumb nails. It starts at the cuticle and grows out to involve the free edge. The nail will often eventually return to normal but the condition can recur.

Transverse Ridging

TRANSVERSE RIDGING	
Physical signs	**Underlying causes**
Transverse depressions	Previous illness (Beau's lines) Chronic eczema Trauma Raynaud's disease Carpal tunnel syndrome
Fine transverse grooves	Chronic paronychia

Transverse depressions which are sometimes slightly elevated proximally are called eponymously "Beau's lines". They were considered by him to be retrospective indicators of a number of disease states. They appear some weeks after an illness or fever and grow out with the nail. The condition is sometimes seen in neonates and marks the transition from intrauterine to extrauterine life.

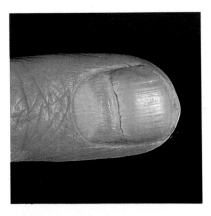

A Beau's line

Transverse depressions in the nail may also be secondary to chronic eczema around the nail fold or they may occur as a result of injury, Raynaud's disease or carpal tunnel syndrome. **Fine transverse grooves** starting proximally occur in chronic paronychia, which is usually the result of a yeast infection.

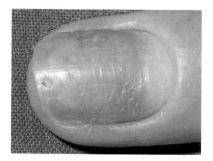

Chronic paronychia showing loss of the cuticle and fine transverse depressions

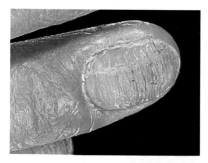

Eczema showing transverse depressions

Trauma to the nail, either occupational (eg. tile fixers) or deliberate, can cause quite marked **transverse grooves** parallel to the proximal fold. They may also be seen in patients who obsessionally push back the cuticle of the nail,usually the thumb nail, either with the opposite thumb or with an instrument, for example those sometimes found in manicure sets. This problem is sometimes seen as a habit analogous to nail biting and the patient is often unaware that he or she is doing it.

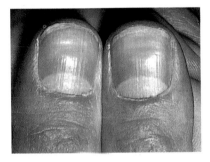

Occupational trauma (tile fixer) showing marked transverse grooves

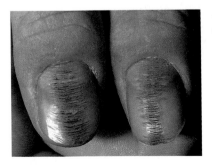

Self-inflicted transverse ridges with ingrained dirt.

Transverse Layering or Lamellar Nail Splitting

This frequent abnormality describes splitting of the distal portion of the nail into layers. It is commonly seen in housewives and others who frequently immerse their hands in water.

TRANSVERSE LAYERING / LAMELLAR NAIL SPLITTING
Underlying causes
Trauma Wet occupation

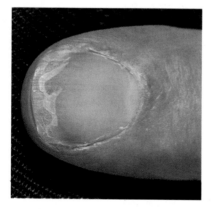

Lamellar nail splitting

Thickening of the Nail

Thickening or hypertrophy of the nail plate can be acquired as a result of dermatological or systemic disease, or may be congenital.

THICKENING OF THE NAIL
Underlying causes
Onychogryphosis
Psoriasis
Lichen planus
Dermatophyte infection
Congenital pachyonychia

Onychogryphosis is usually an acquired abnormality of the toenails seen most frequently in the elderly. It often results from the long term use of ill-fitting footwear and neglect. The big toe is most often involved. The nail is very difficult to cut and eventually grows into a large horny protuberance. Secondary mould infection can occur in this condition.

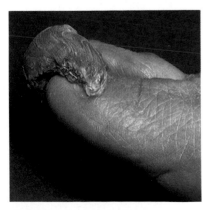

Onychogryphosis

Psoriasis, lichen planus and other skin conditions, when they affect the nail, ultimately lead to thickening of the nail plate. Other signs of these disorders should be sought on the skin surface. Psoriasis causes a number of different nail abnormalities which are discussed in this chapter under the headings of relevant physical signs. Lichen planus is much less common although it produces a variety of nail changes.

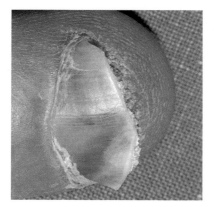

Thickening of the nail due to psoriasis

Dermatophyte infection, which begins distally, results in thickening of the nail plate which starts on the underside of the nail and has a soft friable texture; eventually the whole of the nail plate becomes affected and crumbles away.

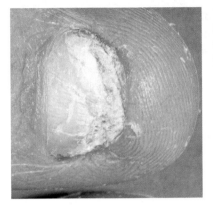

Thickening and disintegration of the nail due to dermatophyte infection

Congenital pachyonychia is an autosomal dominant condition which causes thickening of the nail plate. The fingernails and to a lesser extent toenails become yellowish and extremely hard. Similar congenital changes sometimes affect only the great toenails. The diagnosis should be considered in patients presenting with thickening of the nails in early childhood. In addition to the nail changes a variety of other abnormalities have been described including palmar and plantar hyperkeratosis, warty lesions on the limbs and bullae of the feet.

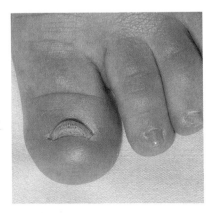

Thickening of the nail due to congenital pachyonychia

Separation of the Nail Plate

Normal nail is translucent and its pink colour is provided by the nail bed. The distal free edge of the nail appears white because of air beneath it and if the nail becomes separate from the bed the white colour will extend down the nail. This change is known as onycholysis and is a common, early presenting feature of nail disease. Sometimes the space between the plate and nail bed fills up with dirt and infecting organisms which leads to further black or green discolouration.

SEPARATION OF THE NAIL PLATE	
Common causes	Minor trauma
	Psoriasis
	Dermatophyte infection (distal)
	Candidosis (proximal)
Less common causes	Photosensitivity
	Circulatory disorders
	Endocrine disease
	Pregnancy
	Syphilis
	Iron deficiency anaemia
	Carcinoma of the lung

Onycholysis commonly results from repeated **minor trauma** to the underside of the nail. It is seen in females who have long fingernails. As a result of leverage, upward pressure is exerted on the underside of the nail which slowly and progressively becomes separated from the bed. The patient will sometimes not present until the condition is well advanced, preferring instead to cover the discolouration with nail varnish. Onycholysis can also occur in men, secondary to occupational trauma but this is less frequent if the nails are kept short.

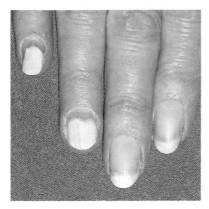

Onycholysis due to minor trauma (note length of nails)

Psoriasis is another condition which leads to onycholysis. It can usually be recognised because the nails also contain small pits.

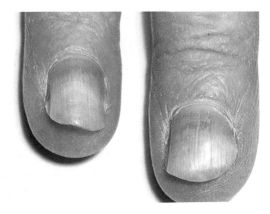

Onycholysis due to psoriasis

Dermatophyte infection of the nails causes a distal onycholysis whilst **candidosis** of the nails secondary to a paronychia can lead to a proximal onycholysis.

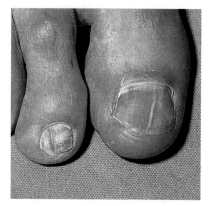

Onycholysis due to dermatophyte infection

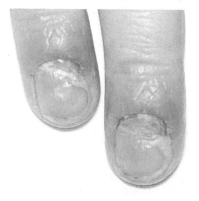

Proximal onycholysis due to *Candida*

Other less common causes of onycholysis include photosensitivity, circulatory disorders, endocrine disease, pregnancy, syphilis, iron deficiency anaemia and carcinoma of the lung.

Discolouration

A number of drugs, chemicals and other physical agents can modify the normal colour of the nail and may be applied therapeutically, deliberately or accidentally. Naturally-acquired nail discolouration is usually white, black, green or yellow.

DISCOLOURATION	
Colour	**Underlying causes**
White	Trauma
	Severe stress
	Cardiac disease
	Gastrointestinal disease
	Renal disease
	Surgery
	Infectious diseases
	Autoimmune disease
	Neoplasia
	Metabolic disorders
	Psoriasis
	Dermatophyte infections
Black or dark brown	Naevi
	Trauma
	Melanoma
	Fungal infection
Green	*Pseudomonas* infection
	Candidal infection
	Aspergillus infection
Yellow	Candidal infection
	Slow growth
	Yellow nail syndrome
	Drug effects

Whitening of the nails or **leukonychia** can be divided into two main types: true leukonychia where the nail plate is discoloured or apparent leukonychia resulting from onycholysis or involvement of the tissue beneath the nail.

True leukonychia may be congenital or acquired as a result of exogenous or endogenous factors. It may be total, striate or punctate. In the striate form the striae may be transverse or longitudinal. Over enthusiastic manicuring can produce both punctate and transverse striate leukonychia. Endogenous leukonychia can result from severe stress and cardiac, gastrointestinal or renal disease. It is also associated with surgery and various infectious diseases. Autoimmune conditions, neoplasia and metabolic disorders may also result in white nails.

In general there is very little disturbance to the integrity of the nail plate in leukonychia. Psoriasis and some dermatophyte infections, namely those due to *Trichophyton mentagrophytes* also cause whitening.

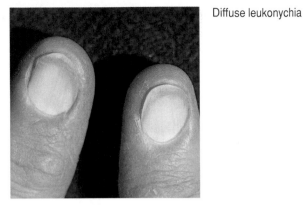

Diffuse leukonychia

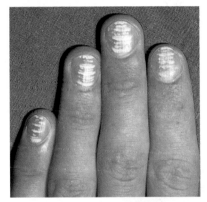

Transverse leukony-
chia

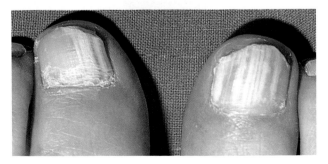

Longitudinal white streaks due to dermatophyte infection

Black or dark brown discolouration of the nails may result from melanin deposition within the nail or from blood collecting beneath it. Naevi originating in the area of the matrix can cause a dark longitudinal streak to appear on the nail. When such naevi occur in adults a biopsy should always be undertaken to exclude a melanoma although they are usually benign. Similarly black discolouration beneath the nail plate should not automatically be diagnosed as resulting from bleeding due to trauma because it is a serious mistake to miss a melanoma in such a situation. Any patient with blackening of the nail without a history of trauma and without evidence of the black area growing out should be referred for specialist opinion.

Some fungi, notably *Hendersonula* and *Scopulariopsis* can cause black, grey or brown discolouration of nails and such discolouration is also occasionally seen in *Trichophyton rubrum* infection.

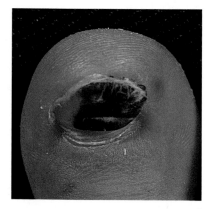

Subungual haematoma

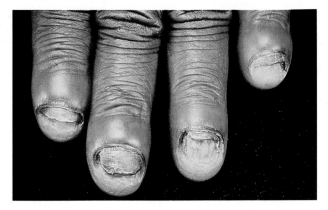

Black discolouration of nails due to *Hendersonula toruloidea*

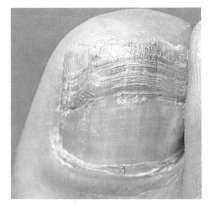

Greyish-black dis-
colouration due to
*Scopulariopsis brevi-
caulis*

Green nails are characteristic of infection with *Pseudomonas, Candida* and *Aspergillus. Pseudomonas* produces pigments such as pyocyanin and fluorescein. The former is soluble in water and chloroform and the latter in water only. Neither *Candida* nor *Aspergillus* produce soluble pigment. A definitive diagnosis can thus be made if the affected portion of nail is soaked in water or chloroform. If the solvent turns green it is indicative of a current or past infection with *Pseudomonas* which can be confirmed by culture.

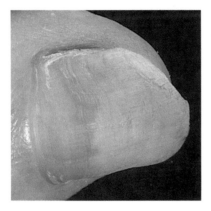

Green discolouration due to *Pseudomonas* beneath a lytic nail

Yellow nails can occur in candidal infection and also as a result of slow growth, particularly in the yellow nail syndrome which sometimes is associated with lymphatic abnormalities. Drugs such as tetracyclines can also cause yellow discolouration of nails.

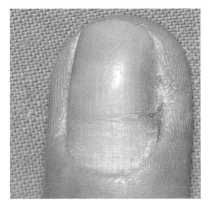

Yellow nail syndrome

Inflammation of the Nail Fold

Inflammatory change affecting the proximal and lateral nail folds is regularly seen in dermatological disorders which affect the fingers. The inflammation may be primary or secondary to separation of the nail fold from the nail plate caused by swelling. This separation leads to infection in the periungual tissues which in turn makes the inflammation worse. Any chronic inflammatory change in the nail folds will tend ultimately to disrupt the nail plate and changes described previously such as transverse ridging or separation of the nail plate can occur.

INFLAMMATION OF THE NAIL FOLD

Underlying causes

Acute paronychia
Chronic paronychia
Eczema
Plaque psoriasis
Pustular psoriasis
Sarcoidosis
Collagen disorders

Acute paronychia is a well recognised bacterial infection, usually due to *Staphylococcus aureus*, which is extremely painful and eventually points and discharges pus. When pointing occurs a small incision can be made allowing the pus to discharge. This generally leads to rapid resolution of the infection. Acute paronychia itself does not cause disruption of the nail plate although an incorrectly sited drainage incision can.

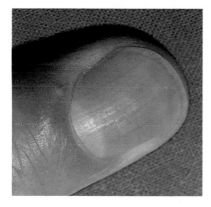

Acute paronychia

Chronic paronychia results from separation of the cuticle which thus loses its waterproof properties and allows infection to wash beneath it. This causes swelling of the nail fold and further separation of the cuticle, which eventually causes disruption to the nail plate. Various bacteria and yeasts of the *Candida* species are usually involved.

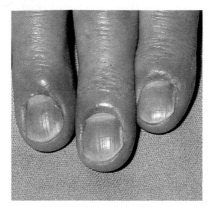

Inflammation due to early chronic parony-chia

Eczema of the distal area of the fingers produces similar changes. There is swelling of the tissues of the nail fold which results in a secondary paronychia. Such changes can occur in all forms of eczema and also in infants who suck their thumbs.

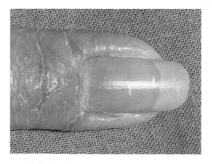

Inflammation due to eczema

Plaque psoriasis, if it affects the distal area of the fingers or toes, can appear inflammatory and also give rise to a **secondary paronychia**.

Pustular psoriasis (acropustulosis) occurs mainly on the palms or soles but can affect the fingertips. It results in sterile pustules developing around and sometimes beneath the nail plate. These pustules initially appear a creamy-white colour which is distinct from the yellow colour of bacterial pus and as they resolve they tend to leave hard brown macules which are of diagnostic appearance. When severe it can lead to complete separation of the nail plate.

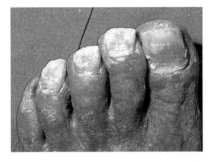

Inflammation due to psoriasis

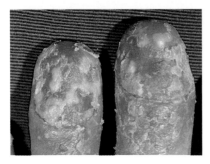

Pustular psoriasis

Sarcoidosis can affect both the nail plate and the nail folds resulting in disruption and fragility of the nail plate together with erythema, scaling and fissuring of the surrounding skin. Splinter haemorrhages can also occur.

Collagen disorders classically cause inflammation of the proximal nail fold. To the naked eye, this manifests itself as erythema of the nail fold, but examination with a good hand lens will reveal tiny telangiectatic vessels which are almost diagnostic of collagen disease, particularly when taken in conjunction with other skin and systemic changes. The nail plate is rarely disturbed in these conditions.

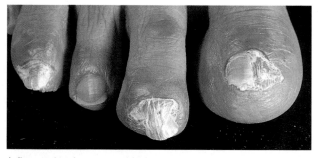

Inflammation due to sarcoidosis

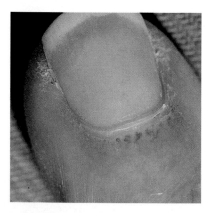

Nail fold telangiectasia

Painful Nails

Pain or discomfort is a subjective sensation and given the rich sensory innervation of the fingertips it can be a presenting symptom of almost any nail disorder. In general however, trauma, inflammation and tumours are the commonest causes of pain affecting the nail apparatus, in addition that is to acute paronychia.

PAINFUL NAILS	
Causes	**Examples**
Trauma	Subungual haematoma Ingrowing toenail
Acute or chronic inflammation	Paronychia Acropustulosis Herpetic whitlow
Tumours	Melanoma Subungual fibromata Glomus tumour

Trauma to the nail is often very painful especially when it results in a subungual haematoma. Direct trauma from the nail itself as in an ingrowing toenail also causes extreme discomfort.

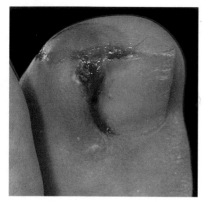

Ingrowing toenail

Acute or chronic inflammation of the nail folds or the nail bed can cause pain especially on pressure and this symptom is seen in paronychia, acropustulosis and herpetic whitlow.

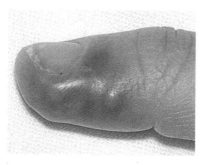

Herpetic whitlow

Tumours such as melanoma, or subungual fibromata are painful when they become large enough or pain can be elicited by pressure. Glomus tumours are almost invariably painful and the discomfort can be severe on occasions.

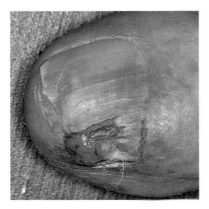

Melanoma

Pitting

Pitting occurs as a result of a defect in nail formation. The surface of the nail becomes covered in small punctate depressions which vary in number, size, depth and shape. Deep pits are associated with psoriasis whereas shallow pits are seen in alopecia areata, eczema, the curious idiopathic condition known as 'twenty nail dystrophy' and sometimes trauma.

PITTING	
Physical signs	**Underlying causes**
Deep pits	Psoriasis
Shallow pits	Alopecia areata
	Eczema
	Twenty nail dystrophy
	Trauma

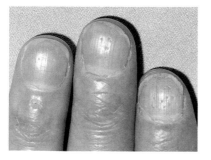

Pitting

Other Abnormalities

There are numerous other visible changes of diagnostic importance which might be seen in the nails. **Splinter haemorrhages** are most commonly due to trauma in which case they are found in the distal portion of the nail. Conditions such as psoriasis which cause onycholysis will predispose to their occurrence. In subacute bacterial endocarditis they can occur in the proximal half of the nail as well.

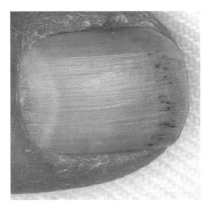

Splinter haemorrhages

Spooning of the nails or **koilonychia,** classically seen in iron deficiency anaemia, also occurs as a physiological variant in young infants. It may also result from thinning of the nail plate from, for example, candidal infection, excessive exposure to detergents, alopecia areata or twenty nail dystrophy.

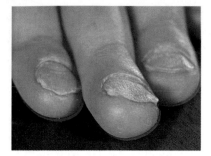

Koilonychia in twenty nail dystrophy

Pterygium is the name given to a change in which the cuticle becomes fused with the nail plate, completely obliterating the nail fold. Most typically it results from severe lichen planus but it is also to be found in graft versus host disease, sarcoidosis and following injury.

The classical sign of **clubbing** is the best known abnormality of nail curvature. It occurs as a result of an increase in the soft tissue beneath the nail fold which causes loss of the normal angle between the nail fold and the nail plate. In addition to cardiac and pulmonary disease it may be an isolated idiopathic finding, sometimes inherited as a Mendelian dominant. Clubbing of just one or two digits may result from a localised arterio-venous anastamosis.

Lateral over-curvature is so frequently seen in the little toenails that it can be regarded as normal. In other toenails it can be idiopathic or the result of trauma or pressure from ill-fitting shoes.

Longitudinal over-curvature or 'beaking' of the nails can result from the loss of soft tissue and is a characteristic feature of systemic sclerosis. Another occasional cause of beaking of a solitary nail is trauma.

Nails may be **shed** for a number of reasons and here again trauma must rate as the most frequent cause, particularly in the great toenails. Severe Beau's lines may cause a complete transverse fracture in the nail plate and the nail may be lost in severe inflammatory conditions such as pustular psoriasis. In the rare nail patella syndrome the nails are absent or vestigial.

TYPES OF ABNORMALITY

POINTS TO NOTE

1. Nails can be affected by many local and systemic conditions.

2. Most nail disorders are not amenable to treatment.

3. Always refer a black or partly black nail for specialist opinion if there is no certain evidence of trauma.

4. Fungal infection is by far the commonest disorder which can respond to treatment and therefore it is very important not to miss it.

Chapter Four

Fungal Nail Disease

Fungal nail disease or onychomycosis is a relatively common chronic infection and a frequent cause of nail deformity. Fungal infection does not normally involve the nails uniformly or symmetrically and can frequently be seen affecting only one or two nails. It can be caused by a number of different fungi, both moulds and yeasts. The majority of infections are caused by moulds called dermatophytes and the infection is variously named either tinea unguium, ringworm or dermatophytosis. Yeasts of the genus *Candida*, notably *Candida albicans* are the second most common cause of nail infection. More rarely moulds such as *Scopulariopsis, Hendersonula* and *Scytalidium* affect nails; these infections are referred to under the general title of onychomycosis and are thought by some to be secondary invaders of previously damaged nail. Although these latter infections are relatively rare it is important that their aetiology is correctly identified since in most cases they respond poorly, if at all, to currently available antifungal therapies.

Clinical Features

Fungal infection of the nail is classified into four different types.

Distal and lateral subungual onychomycosis (DLSO) (Figure 3) affects the distal end and side of the nail and is the commonest type of fungal nail dystrophy seen in dermatophyte infection and also in some secondary mould infections.

Superficial white onychomycosis (SWO) is seen in a specific type of dermatophyte infection caused by *Trichophyton mentagrophytes* and is relatively uncommon **(Figure 4)**.

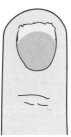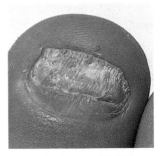

Figure 3. Distal and lateral subungual onychomycosis (DLSO)

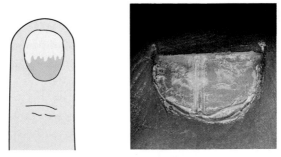

Figure 4. Superficial white onychomycosis (SWO)

Proximal subungual onychomycosis (PSO) arises from the proximal part of the nail and is usually secondary to a chronic paronychia caused by infection with yeasts of the *Candida* species. **(Figure 5)**

Total dystrophic onychomycosis (TDO). This final type of nail dystrophy where the whole of the nail plate is destroyed can be a consequence of any of the first three types. **(Figure 6)**

The clinical appearances of these patterns of infection vary, as do the nails involved.

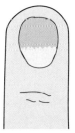
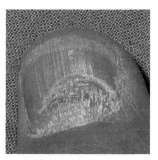

Figure 5. Proximal subungual onychomycosis (PSO)

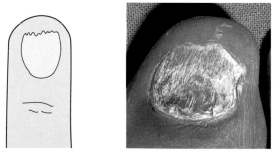

Figure 6. Total dystrophic onychomycosis (TDO)

In **DLSO** the fungus usually attacks the nail through the distal and lateral undersurface, although direct invasion of the nail plate is also possible. The fungus produces proteolytic enzymes which enable it slowly to digest the nail keratin. Initially the nail becomes detached from the bed (onycholysis) thus changing to a creamy-white opaque colour. Thereafter reactive hyperkeratosis develops on the underside of the nail leading to thickening which will eventually affect the full thickness of the nail plate, the top surface consequently becoming ridged and eventually crumbling away. DLSO affects the toenails more than twice as often as the fingernails.

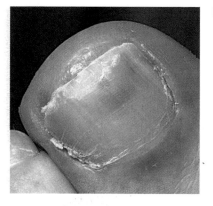

Early DLSO

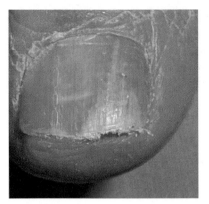

DLSO

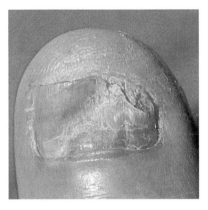

DLSO due to
Aspergillus

In **SWO**, which is associated with a *T. mentagrophytes* infection, the nail plate assumes an obvious white colour. This condition also predominantly affects the toenails but here the site of entry of the fungus is less clear.

PSO is much more commonly seen in the fingernails because it depends upon the cuticle becoming detached from the nail plate allowing the infecting organism to penetrate beneath it. This can be an occupational disease seen most commonly in those such as housewives, hairdressers, nurses and cooks who have a 'wet' occupation. Inflammation of the proximal nail fold precedes this type of nail dystrophy and is often the first cause for complaint. Eventually the proximal part of the nail becomes ridged and ultimately severely disrupted, thus further preventing the cuticle from re-adhering. Hyperkeratosis is not such a marked feature in PSO as it is in DLSO.

It is thus possible to categorise various types of infection on clinical grounds, but a clinical diagnosis should be supported by laboratory confirmation of infection. Certainly therapy should not be started before confirmation of infection because treatment needs to be continued until resolution which may take months. Success or failure cannot be gauged accurately without definitive evidence of infection before the start of treatment. Laboratory confirmation of infection is considered in detail in Chapter 6.

FUNGAL NAIL DISEASE

POINTS TO NOTE

l. Clinical patterns of change in fungal nail disease give a clue to the type of infection present.

2. Dermatophyte (ringworm) infection is commonest, and toe-nails are affected twice as often as fingernails.

3. Proximal fungal infection is nearly always caused by *Candida* and is secondary to paronychia.

Chapter Five

Mycology and Epidemiology

It is important to consider briefly the incidence of onychomycosis and also the origin and types of fungi involved in the different forms of nail infection. However, the pathogenesis of these infections and the host's response to them is a complex, poorly understood area and detailed consideration of these aspects is beyond the scope of this brief text.

The Fungi

There are two main groups of fungi:

(i) **moulds**, where the fungal cells are joined together to form filaments called hyphae which branch to form an interwoven mass, the mycelium, on which the fungus produces its spores; the type and number of spores produced varies from species to species and is the characteristic used most often to identify mould fungi.

(ii) **yeasts**, in contrast to moulds, are predominantly unicellular, usually with round or oval cells. These cells reproduce by a process called budding where a small protuberance develops usually at the poles of the cell; this bud balloons out to form a daughter cell which eventually separates from the parent. In some yeasts the budding cells become elongated and adhere in chains forming what is known as a pseudomycelium. Some yeasts produce true mycelium indistinguishable from that produced by moulds.

A small number of fungi are **dimorphic** and are capable of growth in either the yeast or mould form. The type of growth they produce is dictated by environmental conditions. A number of the fungal pathogens of man are dimorphic.

Very few of the large number of species of fungi are pathogenic to man and animals. Some of these fungi can cause infection in either man or animals, whereas others are species specific and for many of these latter fungi man is the sole host. Infections caused by pathogenic fungi (mycoses) are grouped into three types, namely, **superficial, subcutaneous and systemic**.

Superficial infections, although generally less serious than the others are the most common and account for a great deal of morbidity in the general population. The principal superficial mycoses which may affect the skin, hair, nail and mucous membranes, are: ringworm, caused by dermatophytes; candidosis, caused by *Candida* species; and pityriasis versicolor caused by the yeast *Malassezia furfur*.

Pathogens of Nails

In general those fungi which affect nails, particularly in temperate zones, are specific to man. For the sake of simplicity it is as well to divide nail pathogens into moulds and yeasts.

Dermatophytes

These moulds are the commonest nail pathogens. Although there are some twenty species of dermatophyte, only three species regularly cause infection of the nail and they have the ability to destroy keratin; a property that is fundamental to their ability to affect the nail. Channels and quite large lacunae are seen in the nail plate. These channels are often considerably larger than the hyphae contained within them suggesting that there is extracellular proteolytic enzyme activity, but it has proved difficult to isolate specific keratinolytic enzymes in dermatophyte extracts. It is likely therefore that both mechanical and enzymatic destruction of keratin takes place. Although it is possible to demonstrate both humoral and cell mediated immune responses to dermatophytes and indeed some dermatophyte infections of the skin surface do resolve spontaneously, it is highly unlikely that a nail infection will ever do so.

Dermatophyte infection of nails is associated with athlete's foot. There is a classical pattern of spread of ringworm infection from the skin of the feet, usually the toewebs, to the toenails, groin, hands and fingernails. Therefore, dermatophytosis of the nails is nearly always associated with current or past ringworm infection of the feet. Consequently, its occurrence and spread is associated with the use of communal bathing places and its prevalence, like that of tinea pedis, is highest in adult males.

Tinea pedis and its associated infections are caused by one of three species of dermatophyte fungi, namely, *Trichophyton rubrum, Trichophyton mentagrophytes* (var. *interdigitale*) and *Epidermophyton floccosum*. Most dermatophyte infections of nails, some 85%, are caused by *T. rubrum*, with *T. mentagrophytes* found in around 12% of cases and *E. floccosum* in 2–3%. Occasionally there are mixed infections and also on rare occasions infections caused by other dermatophyte species. The preponderance of *T. rubrum* nail infection probably reflects the persistent nature of skin infections due to this species, its relative resistance to therapy and also the fact that *T. rubrum* is better able to invade nail keratin than other species.

All of these organisms are endemic on the floors of communal bathing places and the incidence of foot infection is high in regular users of these facilities; these include regular swimmers, sportsmen, coalminers, members of the armed forces and any other regular user of communal showers and baths. It is likely that nail infections take a long time to develop, and a history of regular use of communal bathing facilities may be some time in the past. For this reason nail infection is not very common in children and occurs progressively more often into adult life. However, the increasing use of leisure facilities, involving communal bathing by families is leading to an increase in nail infection at a relatively younger age.

Other moulds

Although dermatophytes are the commonest cause of DLSO, (Distal and Lateral Subungual Onychomycosis) SWO, (Superficial White Onychomycosis) and TDO (Total Dystrophic Onychomycosis) there are other assorted saprophytic moulds it is necessary to consider since they account for some 5% of all fungal infection of nails.

Hendersonula toruloidea is a geophilic mould which is a primary pathogen of plants confined to tropical zones. It can however produce disease indistinguishable from athlete's foot and can also affect nails. The pattern of nail infection is as for dermatophytes although *Hendersonula* produces a characteristic black discolouration of the nail because of its intrinsic colour. Whilst not very common it is seen in immigrants to the United Kingdom and occasionally in UK residents who have travelled in the tropics.

Scopulariopsis brevicaulis is commonly isolated from infected nails in the UK although curiously enough it is not often recognised as a pathogen of nails in the USA. This organism is probably not a primary pathogen but invades previously damaged nails and produces a characteristic dark green or grey–black discolouration. Apart from the discolouration, the pattern of infection is again distal and lateral. An experienced mycologist is often able to recognise the characteristic spores of *Scopulariopsis* on microscopy of infected nail material. As with *Hendersonula*, it is important to recognise this organism before beginning treatment because it does not respond to available conventional antifungal therapy.

A large number of other moulds have been reported as causes of onychomycosis and they include *Scytalidium, Aspergillus, Fusarium, Cephalosporium* and *Alternaria* species. They are all uncommon, particularly in temperate zones and are only of importance in that they generally do not respond to conventional antifungal drugs.

Yeasts

Nail infections caused by yeasts are predominantly due to *Candida* species in particular *Candida albicans*. These organisms are common commensals of the mouth, gastrointestinal tract, vagina and to a lesser extent the skin. Estimates vary but it is thought that approximately 20% of the population carry yeasts as a commensal and most infections with *Candida* are believed to be endogenous in origin.

Candida species tend to affect nails in one of two ways; distal nail disease and chronic proximal paronychia. More rarely, *Candida* may cause total nail dystrophy. In distal nail disease *Candida* produces onycholysis and hyperkeratosis which is very similar to the changes produced by dermatophytes. Candidal infection of the distal portion of the nail often produces spooning of the nail which does not occur in dermatophytosis and sometimes such changes are seen in patients with peripheral vascular disease or Raynaud's phenomenon.

A number of *Candida* species can produce such changes and although *C. albicans* is overwhelmingly the commonest pathogen, *Candida tropicalis* and *Candida parapsilosis* often produce disease in the distal nail. There is no definite evidence that yeasts are keratinolytic but given the clinical patterns of disease it is likely that they must at least have some proteolytic activity which destroys the integrity of the keratin.

C. albicans is the predominant organism in chronic paronychia in which it produces chronic inflammation beneath the nail fold and secondarily disrupts the nail plate. Whether or not the organism originates from the patient's own gut or some other body site, or arises from another source, is a matter of continuing debate. However the evidence is that *Candida* species do cause nail disease in both of the patterns described above and would respond to an effective form of anti-candidal treatment.

Chronic mucocutaneous candidosis is a rare form of candidosis in which a specific T-cell defect leads to a diminished immune response to *Candida*. Sometimes this T-cell defect is inborn or can be a result of various endocrine disorders. It is very rare but does cause total dystrophy (TDO) in some nails, usually fingernails, as well as candidosis of the mucous membranes of the eyes, mouth and genitalia.

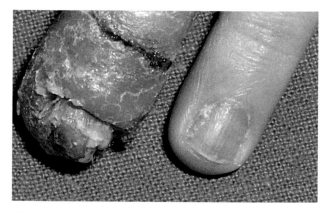

Chronic mucocutaneous candidosis

Prevalence of Fungal Nail Disease

Most UK patients with dermatophytosis who are referred to dermatology clinics show evidence of nail involvement. However, until very recently, there have been no good large scale studies carried out on the prevalence of fungal nail disease in the general population and the only possible approach has been to look at the figures available for the prevalence of foot ringworm and to extrapolate from these. However, most of the studies carried out on the incidence of foot ringworm have been done on at-risk groups of individuals who regularly use communal bathing facilities, such as swimmers, miners, servicemen, industrial workers, etc. It is clear from these studies that the greater the frequency of use of communal bathing places the greater the likelihood of developing foot ringworm (**Table 2**). Coalminers who use communal bathing facilities every day have the highest prevalence.

PREVALENCE OF FOOT RINGWORM	
Group	Prevalence of infection %
Swimmers	8.5
Day schoolboys	8.9
Boarding schoolboys	22.0
Longstay hospital males	39.0
Coalminers	≤80.0

Table 2. The relationship between exposure to communal bathing facilities and prevalence of foot ringworm

There have been few studies of the prevalence of foot ringworm in the general population. It has been shown that among users of a swimming pool, 8.5% had a fungal infection of their feet and that among the male swimmers over the age of 16 the prevalence was 21.5% Another study of office and shopworkers revealed a 14.8% prevalence of foot ringworm. It would appear therefore that 10–15% of the population in the UK could have a fungal infection of the feet. The proportion of individuals with foot ringworm who have a concurrent dermatophyte infection of their toe- or fingernails or both has been found in different surveys to be as high as 30%. It can be assumed therefore that up to one third of those with foot ringworm have some form of nail involvement, and from these data it can be estimated that up to 5% of the general population could have a fungal nail infection.

A recent large survey of the prevalence of fungal nail disease in the general population has been carried out using a questionnaire. Whilst such a study cannot possibly provide information as reliable as laboratory confirmation of infection, its accuracy was first tested in groups with known nail disease and found to be satisfactory. Approximately 10,000 people were asked to complete the questionnaire which contained questions and photographs of different nail disorders. It revealed a prevalence of fungal nail infection of between 2 and 3% in the population surveyed. Extrapolation of this figure would mean that some 1.5 million of the population of the UK are affected by fungal nail disease.

MYCOLOGY AND EPIDEMIOLOGY

POINTS TO NOTE

I. Dermatophytes slowly destroy nail keratin causing the nail to crumble.

2. *T. rubrum* is the commonest nail pathogen.

3. Various *Candida* species can cause nail infection.

4. Some fungi which cause nail disease do not respond to antifungal drugs.

5. Dermatophyte infection is generally contracted in communal bathing places.

6. Dermatophyte infection of the nail is almost always preceded by athlete`s foot.

Chapter Six

Diagnosis of Fungal Nail Infection

Clinical Diagnosis
The pattern of clinical infection of nails tends to fall into one of the four broad groups described on pages 42 and 43, but it is not possible to make a definitive diagnosis of fungal infection on clinical grounds alone. Laboratory confirmation is essential for an accurate diagnosis and also for monitoring antifungal therapy.

Laboratory Diagnosis
General principles
The laboratory diagnosis of fungal infections is based on the examination of clinical material by microscopy in potassium hydroxide (KOH) and by culture. The reliability of these procedures is determined by the expertise of the laboratory staff and by the quality of the sample sent for examination. Nail clippings should be sent to a mycology laboratory experienced in the diagnosis of fungal infections.

Such specialist laboratories are relatively few in number but should certainly be utilised in preference to local bacteriology laboratories unless the latter are experienced in fungal diagnostic techniques. It is a fortunate fact that fungi will remain viable in nail clippings for several months, so sending such clippings to an appropriate laboratory by post presents no problems. In the main, good nail clippings are all that are required to diagnose the majority of fungal nail infections and these are easy and quick to take and can be sent very conveniently to an appropriate laboratory.

Collection of samples

Clippings should be obtained from the affected portion of the nail, taking care to obtain as much of the crumbly material as possible; this material is concentrated on the underside of the nail where the nail is most thickened and therefore a small pair of scissors is useless for sampling purposes. A pincer type nail clipper of adequate size is most useful. As much material as possible should be obtained and folded in small squares of paper (preferably black) or placed within one of the commercial sample transport kits which are available.

Where the nail dystrophy is wholly proximal it is not possible to obtain a specimen by clipping. In such cases a scraping can be taken from the affected portion of the nail with a scalpel blade or material can be obtained by the use of a small biopsy punch. Care must be taken not to cause pain by penetrating the nail. Fungi can be visualised and isolated from biopsy specimens but this requires a local anaesthetic and special expertise in the technique and therefore is not a practical diagnostic method.

Candida can be specifically isolated from beneath the proximal nail fold by running a bacteriology swab dipped in saline along the length of the fold. This allows the saline to wash under the detached cuticle collecting the organism. The swab can then be replaced in its holder and sent to the laboratory. The swab should be processed as soon as possible because if it is allowed to dry out, it will adversely affect the viability of the yeast. The use of a swab sent in plain transport medium prevents this problem. Alternatively, a wire or plastic loop can be passed underneath the nail fold where the cuticle is detached and rubbed directly onto a culture plate but this requires special facilities which are not likely to be generally available.

Laboratory procedures

Once the nail specimen has arrived in the laboratory it is cut into portions of 2–3 mm in size. Part of the sample is mounted in 10–20% KOH on a glass microscope slide, allowed to stand for 10–20 minutes for the material to 'clear' (digestion of the keratin), the coverslip squashed lightly and examined at up to ×400 magnification. The bulk of the sample though is cultured on an appropriate agar medium, usually Sabouraud's agar, and incubated for up to 3 weeks at 28–30°C; when yeasts are the suspected causal agents, incubation may be at 37°C for a shorter period (up to 1 week).

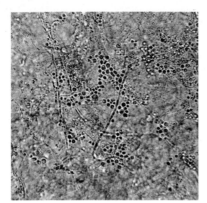

Candida albicans in skin showing yeast cells and mycelium (20% KOH mount)

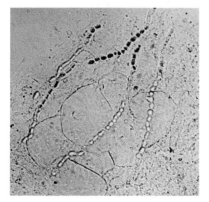

Dermatophyte mycelium and arthroconidia in skin scales (20% KOH mount)

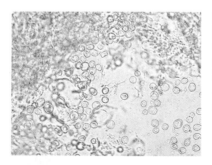

Nail mounted in 30% KOH showing thick-walled, lemon-shaped spores and scanty hyphae of *Scopulariopsis brevicaulis*

Interpretation of results

Recognition of fungal elements in nail is a technique which requires considerable experience and expertise and this is an important reason for utilising a specialist laboratory. Fungal elements within the specimen may be scanty and be missed by the inexperienced, resulting in false negatives. Conversely, cell walls, fibres and other artefacts may be mistaken for fungi and result in false positives. For these reasons, without specific training, it is unhelpful to examine nail clippings in the side room, as the results are not reliable.

Visualising fungal elements by direct microscopy does not identify the type of fungus involved, except that yeasts can usually be differentiated from dermatophytes and occasionally a *Scopulariopsis* infection can be identified by the spores produced in nail.

A reliable identification of the causal agent can only be made by culture. Yeasts grow within 2–3 days and are subsequently identified by biochemical tests. Since most dermatophytes tend to grow very slowly in culture, it is unlikely that the causal fungus can be identified in less than 7–10 days and cultures must be continued for 3 weeks before they are pronounced negative.

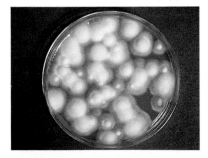

Culture of *Trichophyton rubrum* on Sabouraud's agar showing red pigment at the periphery of colonies at 14 days

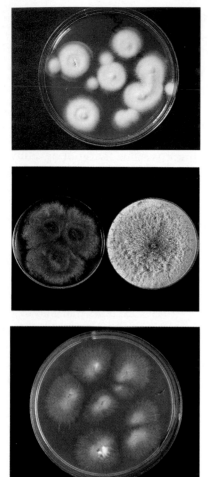

Culture of *Tricho-phyton mentagro-phytes* on Sabouraud's agar at 14 days

Cultures of *Hender-sonula toruloidea* at 14 days on Sabouraud's agar showing two colony types

Culture of *Epidermophyton floccosum* on Sabouraud's agar at 10 days

Any dermatophytes or moulds that develop on culture are identified by the macroscopic appearance of the fungal colonies and by the type of microscopic structures (especially spores) they produce. A definitive diagnosis of the fungal species involved is sometimes of importance in selecting an appropriate therapy. Unfortunately, however, even in the best laboratories, the fungus will fail to grow in culture in up to 50% of nail samples which were positive for fungus by microscopy. This may reflect poor sampling but in most cases it is due to the fact that the fungus in the accessible, distal parts of the nail may be up to 12 months old and consequently is non-viable. If it is essential that the fungus be cultured then a repeat specimen will need to be sent to the laboratory.

Dermatophytosis of nails needs to be distinguished from other mould and yeast infections that may not respond to anti-dermatophyte therapy. Therefore, it is important to identify correctly the species of fungus involved by culture. Nevertheless, it is by and large sufficient to visualise the fungus in nail microscopically in order to confirm infection and institute treatment. Culture results obtained subsequently will serve to confirm the correct choice of therapy or indicate any changes that may be required.

DIAGNOSIS OF FUNGAL NAIL INFECTION

POINTS TO NOTE

1. Nail specimens must be sent to a laboratory with experience in mycology.

2. Nail clippings can be sent by post.

3. Specimens must be taken from the most affected part of the nail with the correct instrument – preferably with pincer type clippers.

4. Looking at nail clippings microscopically in the side room is liable to error, unless the observer has had special training.

5. Ideally infection should be confirmed by a specialist mycology laboratory before treatment is started.

Chapter Seven

Treatment of Fungal Nail Infections

Nails can be treated topically or systemically but in either case the assessment of success or failure should be based upon mycological cure. Because of the nature of the nail plate as a barrier to the penetration of topical agents, systemic treatment with an effective antifungal agent is always likely to prove more satisfactory. The prime function of any antifungal preparation is to eradicate the pathogen, therefore the cure rates quoted here relate to mycological cure. If infection recurs within a short time of stopping therapy, it is likely to be relapse, but if it occurs later it is more likely to be reinfection. More effective fungicidal agents are associated with lower relapse rates than the less effective fungistatic agents. The nail will usually, but not always, return to a near normal appearance once the fungus has been eradicated. Until recently the results of the treatment of fungal nail infections were rather disappointing even after prolonged therapy but clinical trial results with new, more effective anti-fungal agents have demonstrated dramatic improvements in the treatment of these infections.

Topical Treatment

Fungal skin infections, unless they are extensive, are usually treated with topical preparations containing an azole antifungal. There are a number of preparations available in cream, lotion, or spray form but, with one exception, they are not specifically designed for nail infection. The vehicle does not allow adequate penetration of the antifungal agent into the nail and thus they are not recommended.

Tioconazole (Trosyl®) lotion, contains tioconazole as a 28% solution in a penetrating vehicle. It is specifically marketed for nail infection and when used alone is successful in around 22% of cases. It is better used in combination with griseofulvin, a systemic antifungal drug, but even then the cure rates do not exceed 69% and treatment must be continued for a prolonged period. The length of treatment depends upon the rate of nail growth and this is about 6 months in the case of fingernails and 12 months in toenail infection.

Phytex® is a paint containing salicylic acid, tannic acid and boric acid, in a vehicle containing alcohol and ethyl acetate. Little or no information is available regarding its cure rate but it is likely to be much lower than tioconazole.

Monphytol® contains undecenoic acid, salicylic acid and chlorbutol. As with Phytex® little information is available regarding its efficacy but it is also likely to be very low.

An alternative approach is to use an azole antifungal agent in combination with 40% urea under polythene occlusion for 1 week in fingernail infection and 2 weeks in toenail infection. When the dressing is removed the nail is soft and detached from the nail bed. It can be cut back right down to the cuticle without anaesthetic. Application of the mixture is then continued to the growing portion of the nail for a further week or two before allowing the nail finally to grow out. Success rates of around 60% can be obtained using this technique but it is cumbersome, potentially irritant and labour intensive and is not likely to displace systemic therapy other than on those occasions where patients are intolerant of systemic drugs or do not wish to take them. Commercial preparations of such mixtures are not available in the UK.

The topical treatments described above are generally recommended by the manufacturers for use in dermatophytosis of nails. There are no data available on their success rates in other mould infections but they are not likely to be effective. However, removal of the offending nail in such infections using 40% urea under polythene occlusion is an alternative to surgical removal.

Chronic paronychia and candidal infection of the nail plate do not respond well to any currently available topical treatment. A combination of an azole lotion and an antibacterial preparation such as povidone-iodine or sulphacetamide used alternately night and morning is sometimes useful in preventing spread of infection from the nail fold to the nail plate.

In summary, topical antifungal agents are disappointing in the treatment of fungal nail infections. They all require to be given long term, are troublesome to use and offer very poor mycological cure rates. Systemic treatment is a much better alternative.

Systemic Treatment
Griseofulvin

Griseofulvin, a weakly fungistatic agent which is toxic to fungal cell nuclei, has been the mainstay of systemic treatment for dermatophyte nail infections for the past 30 years. It is prescribed in a dose of 1g daily to be taken with meals. It needs to be given for 12–18 months in the case of toenail infection and for 6–12 months in the case of fingernail infection. In fingernails, treatment with griseofulvin is reasonably successful giving around 70% mycological cure rates. In toenails mycological cure rates are only approximately 30%, making it a very disappointing drug especially as it needs to be given for such long periods. Although devoid of very serious side effects, griseofulvin may cause nausea and headache and sometimes these symptoms are intolerable. It also causes intolerance to alcohol and troublesome photosensitivity in some patients. A combination of tioconazole lotion and systemic griseofulvin would increase the cure rates of toenails to 69% but this is still an unsatisfactory total.

Imidazoles

The discovery of azomycin (2-nitro imidazole) in 1955 has resulted in the development of the imidazole, and more recently the triazole, group of compounds. Several imidazoles are available as topical antifungal agents and ketoconazole (**Nizoral**®) can be used systemically. Ketoconazole is active against dermatophytes but its use in the treatment of dermatophyte nail infections is limited due to side effects.

The principal effect of azoles is to inhibit a cytochrome P-450 dependent fungal enzyme system (**Figure 7**) which is involved in the final stages of ergosterol biosynthesis. Azoles may also inhibit the cytochrome P-450 system in the liver and therefore may delay the breakdown of other drugs which are metabolised by the same system. Ketoconazole is occasionally hepatotoxic and this potentially serious side effect limits its use in onychomycosis to infections of the fingernails which have failed to respond to adequate dosage regimes of conventional anti-dermatophyte agents. The treatment of toenail infections is specifically excluded.

New Developments in the Treatment of Fungal Nail Infection

Recent developments in systemic antifungal therapy include a new class of compounds, the allylamines, and a new group of azole derivatives, the triazoles. Preliminary clinical trial results with these compounds have demonstrated a significant improvement over current therapies, in the treatment of dermatophyte nail infections.

Triazoles

The triazoles are the most recent azole derivatives to have been developed. In clinical trials one of the triazoles, itraconazole (**Sporanox**®), has been shown to

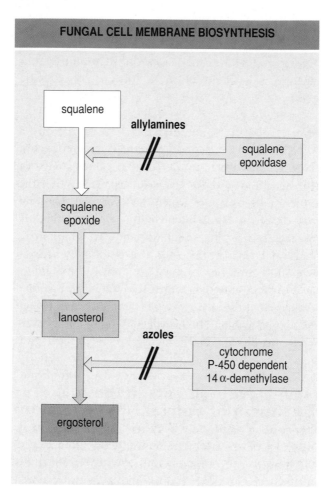

Figure 7. Fungal cell membrane biosynthesis

cure up to 73% of toenails after an average treatment course of 9.4 months, which is an advance on the results obtained with griseofulvin. Data on the treatment of nail infections with the other orally active triazole, fluconazole (**Diflucan**®), are limited.

Allylamines

The allylamines have a different mechanism of action from the azoles **(Figure 7)**. They act by the inhibition of squalene epoxidase — an enzyme which is required for fungal cell membrane biosynthesis. The resulting build up of squalene in the fungal cell kills the organism. One of the allylamines, terbinafine (**Lamisil**®), is available for use systemically. Clinical studies thus far have shown the drug to be dramatically successful in the treatment of dermatophyte nail infections, producing mycological cure rates of 85% in toenails and 95% in fingernails. Moreover, terbinafine appears to work over a much shorter treatment period than griseofulvin (e.g. 3–6 months for toenails) possibly because it is fungicidal rather than fungistatic. Furthermore the relapse rate with this drug appears to be less than that seen for griseofulvin. It is likely that terbinafine will prove to be the treatment of choice for dermatophyte infections of both finger- and toenails. It is as yet unclear whether terbinafine is effective in candidosis of the nail although it does have anti-candidal activity *in vitro*, in particular against *Candida parapsilosis*. In the treatment of other mould infections there is some evidence to suggest that terbinafine may be effective against *Scopulariopsis*, while its effect against *Hendersonula* is not known. However, in comparison with dermatophytes, these moulds are very uncommon.

TREATMENT OF FUNGAL NAIL INFECTIONS

POINTS TO NOTE

I. Local treatment is less effective than systemic treatment.

2. Griseofulvin is only effective in 30% of toenail infections and 70% of fingernail infections.

3. Terbinafine is effective in 85% of toenail infections and 95% of fingernail infections.

Conclusion

Dermatophyte nail infections are more common in the general population than may have been previously thought. With the development of new, more effective antifungal agents, it is all the more important that these infections are recognised. It is hoped that this small book will prove helpful in the identifation and confirmation of nail infections caused by dermatophytes.

Further Reading

Diseases of the Nail and their Management.
Eds. Baran R., Dawber R.P.R.
Blackwell Scientific Publications, Oxford. 1984.

Medical Mycology. A Practical Approach.
Eds. Evans E.G.V., Richardson M.D.
Oxford University Press, Oxford. 1989.

Index

All entries are to page numbers.
Bold entries indicate an illustration.

abnormalities of nails 7–40
  confused with fungal infection 7, 7–36
absence of nails 39
acropustulosis *see* psoriasis, pustular
allylamine antifungal drugs 75
  mechanism of action of **74**, 75
alopecia areata
  koilonychia in 37
  longitudinal ridges in 9, **9**
  pitting in 36
Alternaria, onychomycosis due to 54
anaemia, iron-deficiency
  koilonychia in 37
  onycholysis in 20
anatomy of the nail 3–4, **3**
Aspergillus
  DLSO due to **45**, 54
  green nails due to 26

athlete's foot
  see dermatophytosis, tinea pedis
autoimmune diseases, leukonychia in 22
azole antifungal drugs
  mechanism of action of 73, **74**
  systemic 72–3
  topical 70–2

bacterial infection, in paronychia 29
beaking of nails 39
Beau's lines 11, **11**
  shedding due to 39
black nails 24–5, **24**, **25**, 40
  secondary to onycholysis 18
blood beneath the nail, black nails due to 24, **24**
blood supply of the nail 4, **5**
brown nails *see* black nails

Candida, microscopy of **64**
candidal nail infection 41, 47,
  55–6, 59
  clinical appearance of 20,
    20, 43, **43**
  diagnosis of 61–8
  green nails due to 26
  keratin destruction in 55
  koilonychia due to 37, 55
  onycholysis due to 20, **20**
  in paronychia 20, 29, 56
  PSO due to 43, 47
  route of 4
  sample collection in 63
  treatment of 71, 75
  yellow nails due to 27
  see also yeasts
candidosis, chronic mucocutaneous 56, **56**
carcinoma, lung, onycholysis
  due to 20
cardiac disease
  clubbing due to 38
  leukonychia in 22
carpal tunnel syndrome, transverse depressions in 12
Cephalosporium, onychomycosis due to 54
children
  inflammation due to thumb
    sucking in 30
  koilonychia in 37
  thickening of the nails in 17
circulatory disorders
  koilonychia in 55
  longitudinal ridges in 8
  onycholysis in 20
clubbing of nails 38
collagen disorders, inflammation due to 32, **32**
congenital disorders
  leukonychia 22
  pachyonychia 17, **17**

congenital disorders —*contd*
  thickening of great toenails
    17
cuticle **3**, 4, 6
  fusion with nail plate 38
  loss of, in chronic parony-
    chia **12**
  separation of, in chronic
    paronychia 29
  trauma to, causing trans-
    verse grooves 13,**13**
cytochrome P-450, effect of
  azoles on 73, **74**

Darier's disease, longitudinal
  ridges in 9
dermatophytes
  culture of **65**, **66**, 65–7
  infection by *see* dermato-
    phytosis
  microscopy of **64**
dermatophytosis 41–7, 51–2,
  59
  communal bathing associat-
    ed with 51, 52, 57, **57**,
    59
  immune response to 51
  of nails
    athlete's foot associated
      with 51, 59
    clinical appearance of
      41–7
    diagnosis of 61–8
    keratin destruction in 44,
      51, 59
    leukonychia due to 22,
      23
    onycholysis due to 20, **20**
    route of infection 4
    sample collection in
      62–3, 68
    thickening of nails in 16,
      17

dermatophytosis — *contd*
  prevalence of 51–2, 57–8, **57**
  of skin *see* tinea pedis
  treatment of 69–76
    systemic 72–5
    topical 70–2
detergents, exposure to,
    koilonychia due to 37
discolouration **21**, 21–7
  see also individual colours
DLSO (distal and lateral subun-
    gual onychomycosis)
    42, **42**, 44, **44**, **45**
drugs
  antifungal 69–76
    mechanism of action of
      72–3, **74**
  delivery to nail of 4–5, 6
  yellow nails due to 27
dystrophy
  median nail 10
  twenty nail *see* twenty nail
    dystrophy

eczema
  inflammation due to 30, **30**
  pitting in 36
  transverse depressions in
    12, **12**
elderly patients
  longitudinal ridges in 8
  onychogryphosis in 15, **15**
endocarditis, splinter haemor-
    rhages due to 37
Epidermophyton floccosum
  culture of **66**
  infection of nails by 52
  tinea pedis due to 52

fibroma, subungual
  longitudinal grooves due to
    10, **10**
  pain due to 35

fungi 49–59
  cell membrane biosynthesis
    in **74**
    effect of drugs on 73
  culture of 63, **65, 66**, 67
  dimorphic 50
  growth patterns of 49–50
  infection by 40, 41–7, 50–6
    see also candidal nail
      infection; dermatophyto-
      sis; onychomycosis
  microscopy of 63, **64**, 65
  see also moulds; yeasts
Fusarium, onychomycosis due
    to 54

gastrointestinal disease,
    leukonychia in 22
genetic defects
  chronic mucocutaneous
    candidosis due to 56
  clubbing due to 38
  longitudinal ridges due to 8
glomus bodies 4
  tumours in 4, 35
graft versus host disease,
    pterygium in 38
green nails 26, **26**
  secondary to onycholysis 18
grooves, longitudinal 10
  see also ridges, longitudinal

haematoma, subungual
  black nails due to 24, **24**
  pain in 34
half-moon 4
Hendersonula toruloidea 41,
    53, 54
  black nails due to 24, **25**
  culture of **66**
herpetic whitlow 34, **34**
hyperkeratosis, reactive, in
    DLSO 44

hypertrophy of the nail plate 15, 15–17
immune response
    in chronic mucocutaneous candidosis 56
    dermatophyte infection, to 51
infectious diseases
    Beau's lines due to 11
    leukonychia due to 22
inflammation of the nail fold 28, 28–32
    PSO following 46
    shedding of the nail due to 39
ingrowing toenails 34, 34
injury see trauma

keratin
    destruction of
        by dermatophytes 44, 51, 59
        by yeasts 55
    drugs, incorporation into 5
    formation of 3–4
koilonychia 37, 38
    in candidal infection 55

layering, transverse 14, 14
leukonychia 22, 23
lichen planus
    longitudinal ridges in 8, 9, 9
    pterygium in 38
    thickening of nails in 16
long nails, onycholysis in 18–19, 19
lunula 4
lymphatic abnormalities, yellow nail syndrome due to 27

macules, brown, in pustular psoriasis 31
Malassezia furfur, pityriasis versicolor due to 50

matrix 3, 3–4
melanin deposition, black nails due to 24
melanoma 35
    black nails due to 24
    pain due to 35
metabolic disorders, leukonychia in 22
moulds 49, 51–4
    culture of 63, 65, 66, 67
    growth pattern of 49, 64
    infection by see dermatophytosis; onychomycosis
    microscopy of 63, 64
    see also dermatophytes
myxoid cysts, longitudinal grooves due to 10

naevi, black streaks due to 24
nail bed 3, 4–6
nail clippings 62, 68
nail fold 3, 4
    inflammation of 28, 28–32
    swelling of 28, 29, 30
    telangiectasia of 32, 32
    tumours in 10
nail patella syndrome 39
nail plate 3, 3–6
    fusion with cuticle 38
    hypertrophy of 15, 15–17
    separation
        from nail bed see onycholysis
        from nail fold 28
neonates, Beau's lines in 11
neoplasia, leukonychia due to 22

occupation
    trauma associated with 13
    wet
        lamellar nail splitting due to 14
        PSO due to 46

onychogryphosis 15, **15**
onycholysis 4, 18–20, **18–20**
  in onychomycosis 44
  splinter haemorrhages in 37
onychomycosis
  clinical appearance of 41–7
  laboratory diagnosis of 46,
    61–8
  prevalence of 57–8
  sample collection in 62–3
  treatment of 46, 69–76
    systemic 72–5
    topical 70–2
over-curvature
  lateral 38
  longitudinal 39

pachyonychia **15**, 15–17
  congenital 17, **17**
pain in the nail **33**, 33–5
paronychia
  acute
    inflammation due to 29,
      29
    pain in 34
  chronic 4
    Candida in 29, 56
    inflammation due to 29,
      30
    transverse grooves in 12,
      12
    treatment of 71
  secondary to
    eczema 30
    psoriasis 31
periungual tissue, infection of
  Candida in 56
  inflammation in 28
photosensitivity, onycholysis
    due to 20
pitting of nails 36, **36**
pityriasis versicolor 50
pregnancy, onycholysis in 20

PSO (proximal subungual ony-
    chomycosis) 43, **43**, 46
  sample collection in 62
psoriasis
  leukonychia in 22
  onycholysis in 19,**19**
  pitting of nails in 19, 36, **36**
  plaque
    inflammation due to 31,
      31
  pustular
    inflammation due to 31,
      31
    pain in 34
    shedding of nails due to
      39
    splinter haemorrhages due
      to 37
    thickening of nails in 16, **16**
Pseudomonas infection, green
    nails due to 26, **26**
pterygium 38
pulmonary disease, clubbing of
    nails in 38
pus
  in acute paronychia 29
  in pustular psoriasis 31

Raynaud's disease
  koilonychia in 55
  transverse depressions in 12
renal disease, leukonychia in
    22
rheumatoid arthritis, longitudi-
    nal ridges in 8
ridges
  longitudinal **8**, 8–10
    in PSO 46
  transverse **11**, 11–13
    in DLSO 44
    due to inflammation 28
ringworm *see* dermatophyto-
    sis, tinea pedis

sarcoidosis 32
  inflammation due to **32**
  pterygium in 38
Scopulariopsis brevicaulis 41, 53–4
  black nails due to 24, **25**
  microscopy of **64**, 65
Scytalidium, onychomycosis due to 41, 54
shedding of nails 39
shoes, ill-fitting
  lateral over-curvature due to 38
  onychogryphosis due to 15
splinter haemorrhages 37, **37**
  in sarcoidosis 32
splitting, lamellar 14, **14**
spooning of nails *see* koilony-chia
Staphylococcus aureus, in acute paronychia 29
streaks, dark 24
stress, leukonychia due to 22
structure of the nail **3**, 3–6
surgery, leukonychia following 22
SWO (superficial white ony-chomycosis) 42, **42**, 45
syphilis, onycholysis in 20
systemic sclerosis, longitudinal over-curvature in 39

TDO (total dystrophic ony-chomycosis) 43, **43**
telangiectasia of the nail fold 32, **32**
tetracyclines, yellow nails due to 27
thickening of nails **15**, 15–17
  in DLSO 44
thumb nails
  median nail dystrophy in 10
  self-inflicted trauma in 13

thumb sucking, inflammation due to 30
tinea pedis (athlete's foot, foot ringworm) 52
  nail infection associated with 51, 59
  prevalence of **57**, 57–8
  see also dermatophytosis
toenails, ingrowing 34, **34**
trauma
  black nails due to 24
  lamellar nail splitting due to 14
  lateral over-curvature due to 38
  longitudinal over-curvature due to 39
  longitudinal ridges due to 9
  occupational 13, **13**, 19
  onycholysis due to 18–19, **19**
  pain due to 34
  pitting due to 36
  pterygium following 38
  self-inflicted 13, **13**
  shedding of nails due to 39
  splinter haemorrhages due to 37
  transverse depressions/grooves due to 12, 13, **13**
Trichophyton mentagrophytes
  culture of **66**
  infection of nails by 52
  leukonychia due to 22
  in SWO 42, 45
  tinea pedis due to 52
Trichophyton rubrum
  black nails due to 24
  culture of **65**
  infection of nails by 52, 59
  tinea pedis due to 52

tumours
  glomus 4, 35
  longitudinal grooves due to
      10, **10**
  melanoma 24, 35, **35**
  pain due to 35
  subungual fibromata 10, **10**,
      35
twenty nail dystrophy
  koilonychia in 37, **38**
  longitudinal ridges in 8, **9**
  pitting in 36

vestigial nails 39

white nails *see* leukonychia
whitlow, herpetic 34, **34**

yeasts 55–6
  culture of 63, 65
  growth pattern of 50, **64**
  infection by *see* candidal
      nail infection
  microscopy of **64**
yellow nail syndrome 27, **27**
yellow nails 27, **27**
  in congenital pachyonychia
      17